Prostate Health Guide: Get the Facts and Natural Solutions for Optimal Prostate Health

Disclaimer

This book is intended as a reference material, not as a medical manual to replace the advice of your physician or to substitute for any treatment prescribed by your physician.

If you are ill or suspect that you have a medical problem, we strongly encourage you to consult your medical, health, or other competent professional before adopting any of the suggestions in this book or drawing inferences from it. If you are taking prescription medication, you should never change your diet (for better or worse) without consulting your physician, as any dietary change may affect the metabolism of that prescription drug.

This book and the author's opinions are solely for informational and educational purposes.

The author specifically disclaims all responsibility for any liability, loss, or risk, personal or otherwise which is incurred as a consequence, directly or indirectly, of the use and application of any of the contents of this book.

Individual results may vary.

Published by:
Nick Stanton and Random Technologies
4409 HOFFNER AVENUE, SUITE 347
Belle Isle, FL 32812
Website: http://www.MensGrowth.com

Introduction

Prostate Overview

The Effect of Diet on the Prostate

The Importance of Prostate Health Supplements

Obesity Can Lead to Prostate Cancer

Hydration for Good Health

Exercises for Healthy Living

Treatment Options for Prostate Cancer

Post-Surgery Prostate Complications

Resources

Prostate Overview

The prostate is a gland surrounding the urethra, located in front of the rectum below the bladder.

A healthy prostate is approximately the size and shape of a chestnut and plays a vital role in the male reproductive system.

Its purpose is to produce and release a fluid that makes up a significant portion of seminal fluid. The remaining fluid is produced by seminal vesicles.

These fluids combine and transport sperm through the urethra (the same tube that passes urine) during ejaculation. Seminal fluid neutralizes the vagina's naturally acidic environment, optimizing conditions for fertilization.

Without the prostate, fertility is lost and erectile dysfunction (ED) is common.

Three Main Problems Affecting the Prostate:
1. **Infection**
2. **Enlargement**
3. **Cancer**

All three can cause the following symptoms due to the prostate's proximity to the urethra and bladder.

However, some men who develop prostate cancer will be asymptomatic:
- ☐ Frequent and/or urgent need to urinate
- ☐ Painful urination

- ☐ Blood in urine
- ☐ Awakening repeatedly at night to urinate
- ☐ Difficulty urinating
- ☐ Weak urinary stream
- ☐ Loss of urinary control

Other Symptoms:
- ☐ Sexual dysfunction
- ☐ Pain in the testicles, perineum, lower abdomen, lower back, and during intercourse
- ☐ Fever
- ☐ Sensation of rectal fullness

Over the next few pages, each of these three main prostate problems is examined.

ONE: Prostate Infection

Inflammation of the prostate, or prostatitis, differs in severity, duration and ease of treatment. Of the three main problems afflicting the prostate, infection is the one most likely to affect young men, including teens.

The cause is often unknown, although bacteria found in urinary infections is sometimes the culprit. It is also believed that microorganisms such as Chlamydia can infect the prostate. However, prostate infection from microorganisms is difficult to diagnose.

Another possible cause is untreated prostate enlargement. When there is no apparent cause, doctors commonly prescribe antibiotics, which rarely provide relief when evidence of bacteria is absent.

In addition to bed rest, doctors may recommend vitamins, supplements, plenty of fluids, sitz baths and prostate massage (but not when an acute infection is present).

A sitz bath involves sitting in shallow water, alternating between hot and cold water, and ending with the cold.

Prostate massage requires a willing partner and a relaxed patient. Consult a physician on how to do this safely and correctly.

TWO: Prostate Enlargement

This condition is called Benign Prostatic Hyperplasia (BPII). It is especially common in older men.

As a man ages, his prostate naturally enlarges due to an increase in a hormone called Prolactin. As a result, a chain reaction occurs: an increase in an enzyme known as 5-

Alpha reductase, which leads to an increase in testosterone metabolism, followed by an increase of a metabolic byproduct known as di-hydro-testosterone (DHT). DHT stimulates prostate cells to multiply, eventually leading to prostate enlargement.

This process starts around age 40 and at least 50% of men at age 60 are affected by BPH. 80% of 80 year-old men suffer from this condition.

Though benign, BPH negatively affects quality of life and increases the risk of developing prostate cancer.

THREE: Prostate Cancer

This disease plagues a large percentage of men, especially those over the age of 50.

Approximately 40% of men over the age of 50 are found to have prostate cancer. It is frequently unnoticed and contained within the prostate rather than spreading throughout the body.

In men ages 80-89, autopsies reveal about 67% had prostate cancer. This is typically a slow growing tumor.

There Are Two Important Tests to Determine Risk for Developing Prostate Cancer

1. The first is a digital rectal exam. A doctor inserts one finger into the rectum, allowing him or her to examine the prostate. He or she will be feeling for abnormalities in size, shape, or firmness. A normal prostate is about 2-4 cm long with a triangular shape and has a consistency similar to rubber.

2. The second is the prostate-specific antigen (PSA) test. Those with high PSAs may have a greater risk of developing cancer, but men with BPH may also test high. High levels do not necessarily indicate cancer and low levels do not guarantee an absence of risk. The PSA test measures the level of protein produced by the prostate gland. A doctor will take a blood sample for laboratory testing. This test is sometimes called a biological marker for cancer tumors. Most men normally have low levels of PSA in their blood. If the rate is high, it could point to prostate cancer but it can also mean other non-cancer conditions are present in the prostate.

NOTE: While the former test may be awkward and uncomfortable, it can be crucial to good prostate health. The latter is a simple blood test that measures the protein produced by the cells of the prostate gland. Regular screenings can help avoid the hardships that often befall men who undergo various cancer treatments.

These include:
- ☐ Hormonal therapy
- ☐ Radiation
- ☐ Brachytherapy (small, radioactive seeds implanted in the tumor)
- ☐ Surgery

Prevention is the Best Medicine!
Prevention of prostate problems is the best way to maintain a high quality of life. Many natural, non-invasive actions prevent prostate diseases. Prostate diseases have the potential to interfere with sexual and urinary health. These preventative methods may even prevent loss of life.

Consider this: Don't wait for symptoms to appear

before taking action. Prostate cancer can develop without warning.

Non-invasive means, such as exercise and maintaining a proper diet bolstered with various nutritional supplements, are potentially an excellent alternative treatment that preserves libido, fertility, bladder control and vitality.

Education and a healthier lifestyle can lead to a longer, healthier and more fulfilling life.

The Effect of Diet on the Prostate

A healthy diet is an excellent tool in preventing and treating prostate diseases, including cancer. As an added benefit, this regimen prevents many adverse health conditions, promotes weight loss and contributes to an overall feeling of wellness.

FACT: Western countries have a significantly higher rate of prostate cancer compared with Asian countries. As Asian countries adopt Western diets, their rate of prostate cancer increases. The link between diet and prostate disease is now clear and the evidence points to diets high in saturated fat as the largest contributor to prostate cancer.

Foods including saturated fats are red meat (which may raise the risk of prostate cancer by 30 to 40%), dairy products and deep fried foods. These foods also lead to obesity, which can affect the accuracy of the PSA test, delaying diagnosis and treatment of prostate disease. PSA levels are frequently lower in overweight patients, even when disease is present.

What One Chooses to Eat Is Just as Important as the Foods One Chooses <u>Not</u> to Eat.

On a personal note, it has been my privilege to visit the nation of China nine times over the past few years. With each visit, I am amazed at the large number of older people in their 70s and 80s who are full of vitality.

In virtually every major Chinese city, massive numbers of seniors exercise in public parks. Whenever I ask, "How are you so healthy at your age?" the reply is always the same: "I eat healthy foods."

If you have any Chinese friends, perhaps you have already observed they have a deep understanding of the vital link between specific foods and certain ailments. My Chinese friends have often told me, "If you have *this* condition, you need to eat *that* food." In fact, their conviction of the link between diet and health means many would change their diet before dosing on western medicine!

When setting the goal to add healthier foods to one's diet, consider the following:
- ☐ Eat 5 servings of GMO free fruits and vegetables per day. Many are rich in vitamins, minerals, antioxidants (which fight cancer) and fiber. Remember, to avoid constipation, drink more water when extra fiber is added to the diet.
- ☐ Whole grain foods (including breads and fortified cereals)
- ☐ Cold-water fish and fish oils (Be aware of mercury levels in cold-water fish; this problem has grown with the increase in environmental pollution. Smaller varieties of fish may be a better choice. Take a Selenium supplement to counteract the possible effects of mercury.)
- ☐ Soy products (Ensure that the soy product is GMO free)
- ☐ Green tea
- ☐ Broccoli sprouts
- ☐ Olive oil
- ☐ Seeds and nuts such as pumpkin seeds and almonds that still contain the skin – raw and unsalted is best
- ☐ Flax seed (not the oil as it may promote tumor growth)
- ☐ Low fat dairy and other calcium rich foods

There are a number of vitamins and minerals known for

their prostate cancer fighting abilities. Foods containing Vitamin A, Vitamin B6, Vitamin C, Vitamin D, Vitamin E, Beta-Carotene, Calcium, Lycopene, Selenium and Zinc should be included in a prostate healthy diet.

Vitamin A
Found in apricots, lettuce, spinach, chicken liver and other foods, this vitamin has many health benefits including immune function and cell growth support. It is also important to the reproductive systems in men and women and is best known for the role it plays in good vision.

Vitamin B6
This vitamin is essential for a healthy nervous system and has anti-inflammatory properties, specifically for the skin. Found in fortified cereals, chickpeas (also known as garbanzo beans) and nuts.

Vitamin C
Eating foods such as strawberries, cauliflower, grape juice, red peppers, citrus fruits and juices provides multiple health benefits of this vitamin. It promotes healing, a stronger immune system and iron absorption. Vitamin C also blocks free radicals from damaging cells.

Vitamin D
A deficiency of this vitamin leads to multiple problems. It's needed for healthy bones and teeth and cell growth, Vitamin D aids in reducing inflammation. Sunlight is an important source of Vitamin D. Skin cancer is a concern, but mild exposure to the sun's rays is healthy. Found in fortified milk, salmon, sardines, shrimp, cod and eggs.

Vitamin E
This is another protector against free radicals. It promotes

effective cell communication and gives skin added protection from ultraviolet rays. Take advantage of this effective prostate cancer fighter found in fortified cereals, nuts, spinach and other leafy greens and tomato products.

Beta-Carotene

The consumption of spinach, sweet potatoes, carrots, and pumpkin protects cells from free radicals and improves immune and reproductive systems. Foods rich in Beta-Carotene are also another source of Vitamin A.

Calcium

This mineral is found in dairy products, many leafy greens, sardines with bones, sesame seeds and even blackstrap molasses. Calcium promotes strong and healthy bones, proper nerve and muscle function and affects clotting of the blood.

Lycopene

This fat-soluble nutrient gives tomatoes their deep red color. Its health benefits include prevention of cholesterol oxidation (which slows the progression of arteriosclerosis) and it's another free radical fighter. To maximize the benefits, there should be some healthy fat in the diet. Lycopene in tomatoes is enhanced by cooking; the addition of olive oil furthers enhancement. Consider adding a little olive oil to spaghetti sauce. Other foods containing Lycopene are papaya, pink grapefruit, watermelon and guava.

Selenium

This mineral enables thyroid hormone production, fights free radicals and prevents joint inflammation. Nuts, fish, whole-grain wheat flour, mushrooms and garlic are all excellent sources of Selenium.

Zinc

Blood sugar regulation, metabolic rate stabilization and strengthened immune system are some of the benefits of this micro mineral. It also improves sense of taste and smell. Lean beef, oysters and crab contain a healthy dose of Zinc.

The Benefits of Soy

A study on Japanese men found that those who ate tofu five times a week decreased their chances of getting prostate cancer by 65% compared to those who ate it once a week. Those who drank soymilk daily were 70% less likely to develop prostate cancer compared to those who drank none. In in-vitro and animal studies, soy was found to slow the growth of cancer. An Australian study concluded that the consumption of soy lowered PSA levels by 12.7%.

Foods to Eliminate

Totally avoid or at least reduce consumption of some foods to achieve optimum prostate health.

These include:

☐ Alcohol and caffeine
☐ Animal products
☐ Foods high in saturated fat
☐ Processed sugars
☐ Excess salt
☐ Sugar and sugar substitutes
☐ Hydrogenated oil found in margarine, doughnuts, potato chips, cakes, and deep fried foods
☐ Processed foods
☐ Pasteurized dairy foods (consider eliminating dairy)

Good nutrition is just one powerful ally in obtaining and preserving prostate health. A variety of foods ensures the body receives all necessary nutrients.

Combining this lifestyle change with other healthy habits will be even more beneficial to a better quality of life.

The Importance of Prostate Health Supplements

When considering supplements for prostate health, remember to treat them as seriously as any medication. Supplements may interfere with current prescriptions or increase unpleasant side effects.

IMPORTANT: Before starting any new regimen, ALWAYS consult a physician. A doctor should know all current medications, supplements and vitamins taken daily or weekly.

The Importance of Medical Supervision and Supplements

☐ People on blood thinners should not take Vitamin E supplements.
☐ Those with heart or kidney conditions should not take Magnesium without a doctor's permission.
☐ Vitamin C taken in excess of 1,200 mg may cause diarrhea.
☐ A physician should carefully monitor any consumption of zinc over 15 mg.

Discuss with a doctor if supplements such as the following might provide added prostate protection:
☐ **Beta-Carotene**
☐ **Magnesium**
☐ **Selenium**
☐ **Vitamin A**
☐ **Vitamin B6**
☐ **Vitamin C**
☐ **Vitamin E**

☐   **Zinc**

One Healthy Habit at a Time
As these important changes are made to protect prostate health, don't try everything at once. Don't be overwhelmed by a sudden onslaught of supplements and dietary changes.

Try adapting to one prostate-healthy food at a time. Little by little, the consumption of these foods will eliminate detriments to good health. As a result, feeling better can motivate many to continue transforming their eating habits.

A recent study found that the majority of those who participated in one of four well-known diets quit after only a few months. Gradual dietary changes have proven to be more effective and permanent.

What is Healthy for the Heart is Healthy for the Prostate
The research regarding prevention of prostate disease is lacking in comparison to the abundance of documentation on healthy hearts.

FACT: Diets that are heart healthy also promote weight loss and better overall health, strengthening the body's ability to fight prostate cancer. Extra pounds may prevent early diagnosis, as they can lower PSA levels, giving the deception that no disease is present. It can also make recovery from surgery longer and more difficult, with a less hopeful prognosis. Every man should implement a healthy diet to protect his prostate, emphasizing fresh fruits and vegetables. Such a diet will provide the majority of recommended vitamins and minerals.

The Best Source of Cancer Fighting Nutrients

The American Cancer Society suggests that everyone should obtain all vital nutrients from food, although there is some evidence suggesting there is added protection by taking Zinc, Vitamin C and Vitamin E supplements.

That said, many people claim that food loses much of its nutrients due to mineral deficiencies in soil. Preservatives, processing and chemical additives also play a role in depriving food of nutritional value. This makes it difficult to obtain adequate vitamins through food alone. Ask anyone over the age of 45 if they remember how fruits and vegetables used to taste – especially strawberries and tomatoes!

An Aside: Personally, I believe the wisest course is to cover all bases. Therefore, I strive to eat a very healthy diet and, at the same time, take various supplements. With that in mind, let's look at some of the supplements to consider.

Zinc is considered by many doctors to be helpful in treating BPH. Too much Zinc leads to anemia, immune system problems and can be toxic. Zinc should be taken under the supervision of a physician.

Omega-3 Fatty Acids
Studies have shown that some vegetable oils, fish, and nuts containing Omega-3 Fatty Acids are beneficial for the heart and may have the ability to prevent advanced prostate cancer. Adding a few servings per week should make a significant difference.

Glyconutrients
Taking Glyconutrients can benefit those who are deficient in simple sugars. Numerous studies note significant benefits for those who take Glyconutrients. (See

Vitamins and Minerals
The following list contains the recommended dietary allowances for prostate healthy vitamins and minerals (the total amount obtained through diet and supplements combined):
Vitamin A - Between 3,000 and 10,000 IU per day
Vitamin B6 - Between 1.7 and 100 mg per day
Vitamin C - Between 90 and 1,800 mg per day
Vitamin D - Between 400 and 2,000 IU per day
Vitamin E - Between 22.5 and 1,500 IU per day
Calcium - Between 1,200 and 2,500 mg per day
Selenium - Between 55 and 2,500 mg per day
Zinc - Between 11 and 40 mg per day

Scientists find additional discoveries each year regarding the need for nutrients beyond what typically is consumed through a healthy diet.

Creating new, healthier habits is the most beneficial change men can make in improving prostrate health. Learn about vitamins and minerals needed daily and pay careful attention to one's diet.

IMPORTANT: Remember to have dietary variety as many vitamins and nutrients work in harmony with each other. For instance, foods high in Vitamin C help absorb Iron more efficiently. Varying one's diet will maximize the beneficial qualities of food. It is important to form a partnership with a doctor and discuss methods that promote a healthier prostate, which will lead to better overall health.

Obesity Can Lead to Prostate Cancer

Weight and Prostate Health
Unfortunately for 'Big Pharma' (drug companies), prostate cancer's worst enemy doesn't come in a bottle. Apparently, they are ignorant of this fact and want to keep others ignorant, too.

Controlling one's weight, either by losing it or keeping it off, is the most effective way to prevent the development and advancement of cancer.

However, that doesn't fatten Big Pharma's profits. Since weight loss is a difficult challenge for most men, it's better to prevent weight gain in the first place.

Shrink That Waistline
Men whose waistlines measure 43 inches or more have a 50% increased likelihood of experiencing symptoms of prostate enlargement and undergoing surgery. According to researchers at Harvard University, shedding 7 inches around the waist, or approximately 35 pounds, may be an excellent way to prevent and treat BPH.

Below are some strategies for controlling weight:
- ☐ Drink 2 or 3 quarts of water per day
- ☐ Increase fiber intake
- ☐ Reduce fat and sugar
- ☐ Exercise
- ☐ Eliminate alcohol

Water and Weight Loss
Water regulates metabolism, flushes out harmful toxins,

and keeps bowels moving. This is especially important to remember because increasing fiber intake can cause constipation. Increased water also helps prevent conditions connected to prostate enlargement as well as bladder infections, kidney problems and cystitis.

The Importance of Fiber

A diet high in fiber is a diet high in healthy foods such as fruits and vegetables, beans and whole grains. Increasing dietary fiber has many health benefits, including weight loss.

Lose the Bad, Lose the Fat

Not only do saturated and hydrogenated fats, alcohol, and sugar have no nutritional value, they have harmful effects on health. As intake of these substances are eliminated or reduced, the body loses pounds with more ease.

Get Moving!

Biking, swimming, running and walking burns calories. Try alternating exercises for variety. As exercise becomes routine, men feel better and perhaps find that unhealthy cravings are suppressed. Do simple activities like taking the stairs when given the opportunity or walking a few extra steps when parking the car. When free time is available, be active!

Make these lifestyle changes and weight management may not be as difficult as one thinks.

The Complications of Obesity

As discussed earlier, overweight men face a significantly greater danger of developing prostate cancer.

PSA levels are frequently lower even when cancer has

developed, delaying diagnosis. To make matters worse, overweight men are more likely to develop an aggressive form of cancer rather than the slow-growing variety that prostate cancer usually is. When PSA levels continue rising after initial cancer treatment, such as surgery, "biochemical failure" occurs and prognosis is often poor.

Dr. Sara Strom, a researcher and associate professor at The University of Texas at Austin, stated in a press release, "After surgery, a patient's PSA should go back to being undetectable. But if it begins to rise, that is an indicator of progression."

Obese men are at higher risk for biochemical failure. The reasons are unknown but could be a result of poor diet, sedentary lifestyle or hormonal changes. Impeded healing after surgery is another complication affecting obese men. No matter the reason, losing weight is a very wise move to maintain a healthy prostate!

A Prostate Study
About 70,000 men were observed from 1992 to 2003. Each was asked how much they weighed 10 years earlier; those who had lost at least 11 pounds were 40% less likely to develop aggressive prostate cancer than those who had little to no weight change.

The majority of these men were between the ages of 55 and 74 years old in 1992. Their Body Mass Index (BMI) was calculated, which determines one's ideal weight. BMI measures one's weight compared to height. A BMI of 30 or more is considered obese. In 1992, over 60% of the men studied were overweight, 36% were of normal weight and the remaining 14% were considered obese.
44% of the men said they had little variance in their weight over the past 10 years, which was no more than a 5

pound change within that time. 35% reported gaining 5 pounds or more over the decade and 21% said they lost more than 5 pounds. 5,252 men reported being diagnosed with prostate cancer in 2003, but the majority had a non-aggressive form. The risk to those who are overweight from childhood is unclear at this point.

CONCLUSION: Researchers have concluded that the link between weight gain and prostate cancer is apparent – risk goes up with weight gain and down with weight loss.

Start Today!
Avoid the pills, invasive treatments, surgeries, etc. and start proper diet and exercise. Not only is the risk of prostate cancer reduced, overall health will benefit.

Hydration for Good Health

Water composes the majority of the body and is vital to a good prostate and overall health. Most people cannot live more than a few days without water. Every human cell requires it, just as a car needs gasoline to run.

The Importance of Water to the Body's Functions

People need water to regulate body temperature and metabolism, to salivate, for lubrication, for the fluid that surrounds joints and to keep bowels moving, detoxifying the body in the process.

The following contain an amazing amount of water:
- [ ] Brain – 95%
- [ ] Blood – 82%
- [ ] Lungs – 90%

The Dangers of Dehydration

Just a 2% decrease in the body's water composition can lead to signs of dehydration, including:
- [ ] Fatigue or weakness
- [ ] Dark urine
- [ ] Dry mouth (also known as "cotton mouth")
- [ ] Head rushes
- [ ] Thirst
- [ ] Decrease or loss of appetite
- [ ] Dry skin
- [ ] Flushing
- [ ] Impaired short-term memory
- [ ] Difficulty with basic math
- [ ] Trouble reading fine print

More serious dehydration symptoms include:
- ☐ Headaches
- ☐ Nausea
- ☐ Infrequent Urination
- ☐ Decreased sweating
- ☐ Faster heart rate
- ☐ Increased respiration
- ☐ Rise in body temperature
- ☐ Muscle cramps
- ☐ Tingling of limbs
- ☐ Extreme fatigue

Finally, these symptoms indicate risk of imminent death (when 10% fluid loss has occurred):
- ☐ Vomiting (also a cause of dehydration, as fluids are lost in the process)
- ☐ Rapid pulse
- ☐ Pain while urinating
- ☐ Confusion
- ☐ Dim vision
- ☐ Muscle spasms
- ☐ Loss of skin elasticity
- ☐ Difficulty breathing
- ☐ Seizures
- ☐ Chest pain
- ☐ Abdominal pain
- ☐ Loss of consciousness

It is estimated that 75% of people in the U.S. have chronic, mild dehydration despite the availability of sufficient water.

The recommended amount is at least 8 glasses a day. More is needed for hotter, dryer conditions.

Who Needs More Water?

For some people, 8 glasses a day is not enough. It varies from person to person, depending on environment and the amount of fluid obtained through food.

Below are some examples of people who require more water.

Those Living in Hot Climates

The hotter it is the more likely one will sweat. The more one sweats, the more fluid one loses.

Those with an Intestinal Illness

Vomiting and diarrhea lose bodily fluids rapidly and are both symptoms and causes of dehydration. If possible, drink 2 to 3 quarts of water when suffering from an intestinal virus. Those who cannot hydrate their bodies on their own may need to receive intravenous (IV) fluids. IVs can break the vicious cycle of vomiting and diarrhea causing dehydration, which leads to more vomiting and diarrhea, etc.

Those on High Protein Diets

High protein diets can give cause gout – a painful condition caused by the build-up of uric acid. Uric acid forms crystals resembling needles, causing pain in the connective tissues. Increased water intake can flush out the uric acid, preventing the pain that gout brings. Not only is gout painful, it can cause joint damage.

Those on High Fiber Diets

Without added water in a high fiber diet, constipation will occur due to the fiber absorbing the fluid in the intestines. Drink more water to avoid this uncomfortable condition. About 1 cup per 20 pounds of weight is required.

Taking calcium, iron and zinc supplements benefits health. Drinking the necessary water provides about 30% of the calcium needed daily.

Those Who Are Especially Physically Active
Intense exercise can cause the loss of up to 2 liters of water per hour through perspiration. Always replace the fluids lost through exercise.

What's in Water and Can It Harm the Prostate?
The amount of water consumed is important; so is quantity. Prostate cancer has been linked to water contaminants. Water sources cannot always be trusted even though the Environmental Protection Agency (EPA) regulates municipal tap water.

Hold the Atrazine!
The EPA regulates a chemical called "Atrazine," which is an ingredient found in weed killers. It seeps into our soil, eventually reaching our water supply.

The level of allowable Atrazine set by the EPA is based on a yearly average. Depending on the season, one may be consuming dangerous amounts of this chemical.

Bottled Water: Friend or Foe?
It's a common sight - health conscious people toting a bottle of healthy mountain spring water. Unfortunately, many people aren't unaware that they aren't only drinking water but also the chemicals used in the bottle packaging process. The larger the bottle, the worse the exposure. It's better to drink water from the tap (through a water filter) in a glass.

Purifying Water
There are several options available to ensure the safety of

water. Prostate cancer is especially affected by environmental factors and it's important to make ensure that water intake is plentiful and pure. A reverse osmosis filter for the entire house is a good option as even the steam from chlorinated water can be harmful. Tap water can also contain bacteria and metals.

Distilled water is also an option but is not as convenient and may not be as cost effective. A less expensive choice would be a filter for a single faucet. However, filters tend to be cumbersome and need replacement often. Whatever the choice, purified water is healthier and tastes better, giving the impetus to drink more water.

Cancer Treatment and Water
Surprisingly, 70% of prostate cancer patients die of causes unrelated to the disease. Water is of even greater importance for these men as it regulates important hormones vital to their recovery and immune system. Adequate water intake protects against many forms of cancer including colon, bladder and breast - not to mention other diseases.

Remember: Those who are thirsty are already dehydrated. Try to monitor the amount consumed each day to learn what amount is needed. Don't underestimate water's powerful ability to fight prostate cancer.

Exercises for Healthy Living

Exercise is one of the most important activities for prostate and overall health. Many people claim that they don't have time for exercise. However, the time taken for exercise doesn't compare to the full schedule required to fight cancer. Think about the time spent each day watching TV or movies and surfing the Internet. So is there no time available for exercise? Or is it not a priority?

Consider the family's activities. An evening of sitting on the couch together could be replaced with playing ball at the park, swimming, biking together, going for nature walks, etc. Couples can choose health-promoting activities for dates instead of silently sitting in a movie theatre, munching on junk food.
Be creative and have fun! Exercise doesn't have to be a chore.

Killing Two Birds with One Stone
Those who just cannot bring themselves to part with their favorite TV shows can exercise and watch TV at the same time. Below are basic daily exercises recommended by trainers.

These exercises maximize a workout by using a variety of muscles.
- ☐ **Push-ups**
- ☐ **Lateral Pull-Down and Bent Over Rows**
- ☐ **The Plank**
- ☐ **Lunges**
- ☐ **Squats**

Those with a truly hectic schedule can exercise 2-3 times a

week.

Push-ups
A familiar activity, yet some may need a refresher on how to do it correctly. Remember that the hands should be slightly wider than shoulder width.

While on the hands and toes, keep the abdominal muscles pulled in and the body in a straight line with the head tucked in. Slowly lower to the ground, maintaining the correct position. Once the elbows are at a 90° angle, exhale while pushing up. This exercise works the triceps, shoulders and chest.

Is it too difficult? Try them against a wall, which causes the arms to bear less weight. Or do push-ups on the knees. Once strength is built, move to the toes.
Start with 10 push-ups; add one at every new exercise session.

Lateral Pull-down and Bent Over Rows
A lateral pull-down machine is required for this exercise. Should one not be available, do an exercise called "Bent Over Rows" that works the same muscles.

While sitting at the machine, place the hands on the bar a little more than shoulder's width apart. Lean back approximately 10° and pull the bar toward the chin while keeping abs in, back straight and squeezing the outer back muscles. Do this between 12-16 times for maximum benefit.

This exercise works the abdominal muscles, arms and major muscles in the back, also known as the *latissmus dorsi*.

Bent Over Rows are great to do at home but weights are needed. They are a great alternative to the lateral pull-down exercise.

With the left knee and hand resting on a bench, keep the back straight and parallel to the floor while lifting the weight toward the hip. When the elbow is at more than a 90° angle, straighten the arm and lower the weight towards the ground. Repeat this 12-16 times and then switch sides.

The Plank
This is a Pilates move similar to a push-up. Start with face on the floor and arms at the sides. Slowly push up on the hands, pull in the abdominal muscles, keep the body straight and hold for 30 to 60 seconds.

Repeat this as many times as can be tolerated. Beginners can do this on their knees.

Lunges
This is a great move for the calves, hamstrings, glutes, and quads.

Stand with one leg forward and one leg back. Bend knees slowly until they reach a 90° angle, making sure to keep weight on the heels. Important note: Do not allow the knees to go past the toes or lock them when coming back up.

Do about 12-16 repetitions.

Squats

This exercise also works the calves, glutes, hamstrings, and quads.

Stand with feet about as wide as the hips. While keeping the toes pointing straight in front or slightly outward, slowly lower as if sitting on a chair.

Continue until thighs are parallel with the floor and knees are at a 90° angle. Remember to keep the abs in and the torso straight while not allowing the knees go past the toes.

The Benefits of Exercise

All of the above exercises have tremendous benefits, including calorie burning, muscle strengthening and improvement of balance. Best of all, they take little time and are another way to keep the prostate healthy. Include cardiovascular exercise such as walking, running, biking, aerobics and swimming.

A Word about Biking: Some people believe it can cause prostate infection; however, it seems to do just the opposite.

Have a neglected exercise bike, treadmill or other piece of exercise equipment? Dust them off and make them useful again! Whatever the choice, commitment to a more active lifestyle is vital to health and survival.

Make this goal a top priority. People who exercise feel better, manage weight easier and perhaps find new activities to enjoy with friends and loved ones.

Treatment Options for Prostate Cancer

When a patient is diagnosed with prostate cancer, physicians may become solely focused on eradicating the disease. They may overlook adverse side effects or the fact that only 1 in 8 men will become terminally ill from the malignancy.

Should the doctor's only goal appear to be eradicating prostate cancer from the patient's body, consider changing practitioners.

The wait and see approach, known as "surveillance therapy" is controversial as there is no guarantee of being one of the fortunate seven with a less aggressive cancer and the ability to manage it through natural means.

Patients should strongly consider closely monitoring the rate of their tumor growth. This vigilance will help preserve their quality of life. There is always the option of choosing conventional treatments later if it becomes apparent that their lives are at stake.

Some men decide to enjoy their remaining years rather than suffer through the possible trials of incontinence and impotency. Many men have opted for surgery, radiation and other invasive treatments only to find that their quality of life suffers. Even worse – the cancer often returns.

Consider the following while weighing the pros and cons of conventional treatments.

Statistics Regarding Prostate Cancer Treatment

Each year, approximately 40,000 men have almost immediate surgical treatment or radiation when they are diagnosed with prostate cancer – frequently within 48 hours.

☐   Within 5 years, 35% of these men will have a recurrence.
☐   Within 10 years, 62% will see their cancer return.

Some patients may decide to live at all costs. Others may opt for a possible shorter life, but one with better quality.

Valuable References

The following articles may be a great help when deciding between treatment options:

Prostate Biopsies Risky and Unnecessary. From *Life Extension Foundation,* Ralph Moss, PhD. This discusses complications, including how a biopsy might even enable spreading the cancer.
www.pheonixsonograms.com/risks-of-biopsies.html

Prostate Surgery Has 35% Relapse Rate in 5 Years From *Medical Tribune.* This is an informative article explaining why prostate surgery is frequently repeated.
www.prostate90.com/conven_treat/35relapse.html

Prostate Surgery Has 75% Relapse Rate in 10 Years From *The Urologic Clinics of North America.* More information on the complications of surgery.
www.prostate90.com/conven_treat/75relapse.html

The Causes of Prostate Cancer--The Medical View Contains an overview of the relationship between vasectomy and prostate cancer. It also cites a study featuring the lower incidence of prostate cancer in Mormon men who abstain from cigarettes and alcohol.
www.prostate90.com/conven_treat/caus_pro_can.html

When Disease Recurs...Diagnosis and Treatment Options. By Dr. Guy Bernstein, Urologist at Byrn Mawr Hospital. This article includes helpful information on the common side effects of conventional cancer treatments.
www.prostate90.com/conven_treat/disease_recurs.html

European Study of Effectiveness of Hormones and Radiotherapy Combined From the *New England Journal of Medicine* – Discusses the possible benefits of these treatments.
www.prostate90.com/conven_treat/eff_hor_rad.html

Making the Decision
Whatever the decision, ensure that the doctor supports the patient's wishes and keeps holistic health and well-being in mind. A physician who is completely honest about the impact of the preferred plan of action is of great benefit to the patient.

Post-Surgery Prostate Complications

Prostate surgery and other treatments may cause multiple life-altering complications. They include:

Loss of Fertility
One of the most devastating trials associated with prostate surgery is the inability to father children through sexual intercourse.

While it is still possible to achieve orgasm (in this case "dry orgasm" – so-called because ejaculation no longer occurs), the removal of the prostate and nearby seminal vesicles makes it impossible for sperm to travel to the egg due to the absence of semen.

Fertility is usually impaired by radiation, as the semen produced following this procedure tends to transport the sperm inadequately.

Fertility Options
Should one decide to undergo a prostatectomy (prostate removal) or radiation, it is often recommended that the patient consider "sperm banking" – a process that involves freezing healthy sperm prior to treatment.

After being frozen in liquid nitrogen, approximately 50% of the sperm will survive after they are thawed. Men who want children later in life should consider this option. Storing three to four samples is recommended and they can be frozen indefinitely.

Another option is extracting the sperm directly from the

testicles. This procedure is only possible if the testicles have not been negatively impacted by radiation. It has a somewhat low success rate. An egg is injected with sperm and, if an embryo forms, it is then implanted into the woman's womb. This is known as intracytoplasmic sperm injection.

In addition to being relatively invasive, these procedures are expensive as well. Due to men waiting longer in life to have children and, subsequently diagnosed at a younger age with prostate cancer, there has been an increase in male infertility.

Erectile Dysfunction

Due to nerve damage, many men have trouble achieving or maintaining an erection following prostate surgery. Not surprisingly, this is a very upsetting outcome for the patient and one that is embarrassing to discuss, even with one's partner.

Rather than discuss the problem, many men will simply avoid intimacy to hide the fact that they are suffering from ED.

There are treatments that are sometimes successful in dealing with erectile dysfunction following prostate surgery, but there are no guarantees.

Open communication with one's physician regarding this probability is important.

Loss of Bowel or Urinary Control

Losing the ability to control one's bowel movements or bladder is another unpleasant side effect of prostate surgery. Although it can be temporary, it is often a great source of humiliation and inconvenience. This problem can range from the excretion of just a few drops to the complete emptying of the bladder.

The prostate surrounds the urethra and helps prevent leakage of urine. This is why incontinence tends to develop when the prostate is removed. Radiation can weaken the bladder and decrease its previous capacity. This may also cause uncontrollable spasms that force out urine.

Moreover, the muscles that help control the bladder so efficiently before can be damaged by the radiation.

Men who suffer from incontinence find it necessary to center their activities around bathroom facilities, causing them to avoid activities once taken for granted.

It can also be a danger for older men who have a higher risk of falling. Rushing to the bathroom with great urgency may increase that risk.
There are treatments to counteract the problem of incontinence but it is much easier to avoid surgery in the first place.

Conclusion

The decision to undergo surgery or radiation is one that should be considered very carefully. Researching these options is vital to maintaining a desirable quality of life.

Most importantly, prevention through healthy lifestyle changes will help avoid the many downfalls of prostate cancer and other illnesses.

Resources

Learn More

Visit MensGrowth.com to check out the latest advice for men who are looking to be ambitious... Master their lifestyle... Perform in the bedroom... Experience better health, wealth and personal growth...
www.MensGrowth.com

Newsletter

Sign up to MensGrowth.com newsletter to get strategies for better health, increased wealth, style, sex and personal growth news to your inbox.
www.MensGrowth.com/join